Brain S

A Handbook on Encephalitis

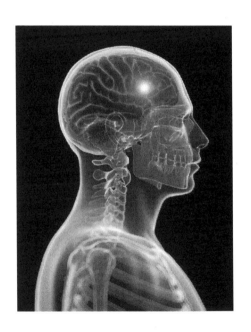

By
Paolo Jose de Luna

Paolo Jose de Luna

Table of Contents

INTRODUCTION 2
What is Encephalitis?..5
Who Are At Risk for Encephalitis? 8
The Different Causes of Encephalitis........10
Signs and Symptoms..15
Diagnosing Encephalitis................................23
Management of Patients with Encephalitis 29
Fact Sheet on Encephalitis 40
CONCLUSION 43

INTRODUCTION

The brain is one of the most important vital organs, possessing the hierarchy of controlling everything about the body from head to toe, up to the involuntary vital organs that we have. Often being compared to the heart, the importance of the brain is never taken for granted as the brain is usually the target of protection when it comes to our daily lives like wearing safety helmets in construction areas and while riding a motorcycle, the body automatically taking defense when the head is attempted to be struck, and more.

There are various types of medical conditions that can affect the brain. This ranges from a simple headache up to a serious tumor growth. However, unlike other medical cases, the standard of practice for treating conditions involving the brain is difficult and demanding since handling the brain is a pain-staking and delicate procedure. That's the reason why healthcare practitioners who care for patients with neurological conditions are highly trained and specialized in their field of practice.

Encephalitis comes from the Ancient Greek words *enkephalos* which means "brain" and the suffix *–it is* which means "inflammation". In other words, encephalitis is essentially the inflammation of the brain. This acute inflammation of the brain often comes from infection, usually viral or bacterial in origin. Nevertheless, encephalitis is considered as one of the most fatal medical conditions in the world that has an incidence 6-8 in a 100,000 population every year. Just in 2013, the estimated mortality rate of encephalitis is found to be around 77,000 which has decreased over the years, but can be still encountered in hospitals, usually in the intensive care setting.

In this eBook, we'll be discussing everything about encephalitis – what it is, what its causes are, its signs and symptoms, the risk factors in developing encephalitis, the methods on how to diagnose encephalitis, and how to manage this life-threatening neurological condition.

What is Encephalitis?

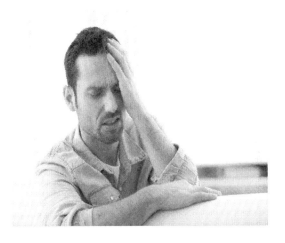

Encephalitis is the acute inflammation of the brain resulting from a viral infection or an autoimmune response in which the immune system mistakenly attacks the brain tissue.

The onset of encephalitis is sudden and develops rapidly. It requires emergency medical care to get a good prognosis for the patient, but those who opt to delay medical consultation often develop a poor prognosis being time as an essential factor in diagnosing and treating encephalitis. This neurological infection can develop from measles, about 1 out of 1,000 cases of measles.

Encephalitis often presents with flu-like symptoms like fever, severe headache, and fatigue. However, neurologic signs and symptoms may also develop like confusion, seizures, problems with sensory and motor functions, and more. But there are some cases of encephalitis that may present with mild or even no signs and symptoms at all.

Severe cases of encephalitis are considered as a life-threatening condition. It comes as unpredictable which makes the diagnosis and the treatment of encephalitis difficult.

Epidemiology

From the statistics of the Center for Disease Control and Prevention (CDC), encephalitis has been found to occur in about 0.5 out of every 1,000,000 people, mostly affecting children, the elderly, and those who have a weakened immune system.

The National Health Service (NHS) in UK has recorded about 1.5 cases of encephalitis in every 100,000 individuals, but officials suspect that this number may be higher since there are many cases that can go unreported when the signs and symptoms are mild.

Onset and Progression

Encephalitis often develops with signs and symptoms that mimic the flu which starts with a fever and a headache. However, these signs and symptoms rapidly worsen even with the use of medications.

More serious signs and symptoms like seizures, confusion, drowsiness, sudden loss of consciousness, or even coma can develop if the person with a suspected case of encephalitis isn't brought in for consultation and management immediately.

Though considered as a serious medical condition, encephalitis is surprisingly found to be rare as a life-threatening condition.

Encephalitis can be divided into two main categories, namely, primary encephalitis which develops from a direct infection of the brain or the spinal column, and secondary encephalitis which can occur from another infection that started off elsewhere in the body and then ascended to the brain which caused encephalitis.

Who Are At Risk for Encephalitis?

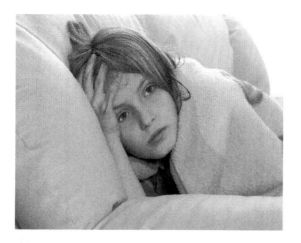

Encephalitis is an infectious condition if proper measures are not instituted. Standard precautions should be implemented for those with encephalitis to prevent further spread of the disease to others. Some groups are considered at risk when it comes to developing encephalitis. These may include the following:

- Children (Especially infants and younger children)
- Elderly (Those above 60 years old)
- Immuno-compromised state (e.g. HIV infection, cancer, etc.)
- Undergoing chemotherapy
- Taking corticosteroids
- Geographic locations (Tropical countries)
- Presence of active infection (e.g. pneumonia, sepsis, etc.)

The Different Causes of Encephalitis

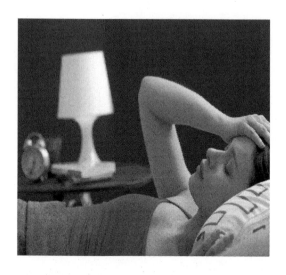

Encephalitis can be divided into various types depending on its causes. The types of encephalitis can be literally categorized into the agent that caused the inflammatory process of the brain and the treatment options also vary for these causative agents. Here are the different types of encephalitis:

Viral Encephalitis

Viral encephalitis is caused by a virus, hence its name. This can either occur from a direct infection to the brain tissue or from the spread of infection coming from another location in the body which may be from the lungs, the gastrointestinal tract, the blood, the heart, and the kidneys. The common causes of viral encephalitis include rabies, herpes simplex virus, polio, measles, varicella, and the JC virus. Other causes of viral encephalitis may include the flaviviruses like the Japanese encephalitis virus, the West Nile virus, the Togaviridae virus, the variola viruses, and more. Finding out what the viral agent that may have caused the encephalitis is essential in determining the treatment options and medications to be used in resolving viral encephalitis.

Bacterial Encephalitis

Bacterial encephalitis can come from a bacterial infection like meningitis that spreads to the brain tissue or a complication from other bacterial infections like severe pneumonia, tuberculosis, syphilis, and more. Other causes may include protozoal or parasitic infections like malaria, amoebic meningoencephalitis, toxoplasmosis, Lyme disease, streptococci infection, staphylococci infection, and other Gram-negative bacteria.

Limbic System Encephalitis

Also referred as "limbic encephalitis", this unique type of encephalitis is where the causative agent of the infection attacks the limbic system. This part of the brain is responsible for the regulation of human emotions and other functions of the body like control of adrenaline, long-term memory, and the sense of smell. Those with limbic system encephalitis often present signs and symptoms associated with emotions such as confusion, irritability, mood changes, paranoia, psychosis, agitation, sleep disturbances, and in severe cases, seizures, delusions, hallucinations and sudden outbursts.

The most common types of limbic system encephalitis include the Anti-Hu limbic encephalitis which is often caused by a small cell carcinoma growth within the lungs, the Anti-Ma2 limbic encephalitis which is associated with germ-cell tumors that start from the testicles, and the Anti-NMDA receptor limbic encephalitis which is a rare, acute form of encephalitis that is highly fatal, but often recoverable condition, wherein an autoimmune response of the body attacks the NR1 subunit of the NMDA receptors, resulting in behavioral changes overtime and recovery from Anti-NMDA receptor limbic encephalitis often leaves the patient with some neurologic deficits.

Autoimmune Encephalitis

An autoimmune response of the body can result in encephalitis. This type of encephalitis can occur from conditions like Anti-GAD antibodies, Anti-NMDA receptor antibodies, and in Hashimoto's encephalitis. Since most of these autoimmune forms of encephalitis don't have tumor growth and the etiology of the condition is unclear, diagnosis becomes even more difficult and it can lead to delayed management and treatment of the condition. Oftentimes, supportive management is the primary intervention given for patients with autoimmune encephalitis as it can regress overtime.

Encephalitis Lethargica

A rare and an atypical form of encephalitis, *encephalitis lethargic* was considered as an epidemic back in 1918 up to the 1930s. Patients who have survived this type of encephalitis have undergone a semi-conscious state that even lasted for decades. Oliver Sacks, a neurologist, used the drug for Parkinson's Disease, L-DOPA or levodopa to revive those who were still alive back in the 1960s.

While there are a few cases of encephalitis lethargic in recent years, the cause is now speculated as a bacterial infection of the brain or an autoimmune attack stemming from an infection. Today, the use of L-DOPA is still the drug in treating those with encephalitis lethargica.

Signs and Symptoms

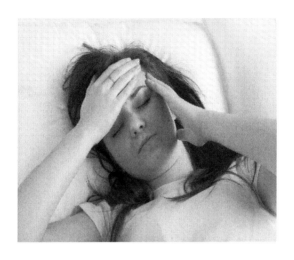

Encephalitis often starts off with flu-like symptoms like fever, headache, muscle or joint pain, and weakness. As the disease progresses, neurologic deficits can be noted like confusion, listlessness, sleep disturbances, psychotic changes, emotional disturbances, seizures, photophobia, and even coma. The signs and symptoms of encephalitis mostly rely on the extent of the infection, the degree of the brain swelling, and the parts of the brain that are affected by the infection.

Because of the infection, the brain becomes inflamed and swells in an effort to fight off the infection. However, since the skull is a non-expandable space, the brain tissue, blood, and cerebrospinal fluid (CSF) become compressed in that area and increase the pressure within the skull. Thus, signs and symptoms of increased intracranial pressure (ICP) may also be present in those with encephalitis.

Other less common signs and symptoms may include those that mimic meningitis (which can lead to misdiagnosis of the condition) like nuchal rigidity, Brudziski's sign, slowing of movements, confusion, fatigue, photophobia, and cough.

Severe cases of encephalitis may also include signs and symptoms like severe and throbbing headaches, confusion, loss of consciousness, high grade fever, nausea, vomiting, memory loss, speech problems, sensory problems, motor function deficits, difficulty in swallowing, hallucinations, seizures, behavioral changes, and even coma.

Brain Set Ablaze

In summary, signs and symptoms that can be seen in patients with encephalitis may include any of the following:

- Headache (throbbing and excruciating in severe cases)
- Fever (high grade in severe cases of infection)
- Muscle or joint pain
- Fatigue
- Confusion
- Weakness
- Agitation
- Hallucinations
- Seizures
- Loss of sensory functions
- Loss of motor functions
- Paralysis
- Double vision
- Photophobia
- Getting unusual smells without stimuli (burnt meat, eggs, etc.)
- Speech problems
- Hearing problems
- Loss of consciousness
- Nausea and vomiting
- Dystonia
- Body stiffness
- Difficulty in swallowing

- Poor feeding in children
- Bulging fontanels in infants
- Behavioral changes
- Psychosis
- Coma

Pathophysiology of Encephalitis

There are several risk factors that put some people prone to the development of encephalitis. Being particularly young or old seems to be a trend over the years in the incidence of encephalitis because the young and the elderly don't have strong immune systems which make them prone to develop encephalitis. Those with a weakened immune system like in the cases of HIV infection or those who are taking drugs that compromise the immune system also put those people prone to getting encephalitis. Geographic locations and seasons also play a role in the risks of encephalitis as there are particular locations and seasons wherein tick-borne and vector-borne viruses are more common.

Encephalitis begins when the brain is attacked by an infection, often viral in origin, sometimes bacterial or fungal, and at times, it may be an autoimmune response of the body which attacks the brain tissue. Once the infection starts in the brain, it activates the inflammatory response of the body wherein the brain swells in an attempt to fight off the active infection.

The defense of the brain against infection (and even other injuries) is one of the strongest defense mechanisms of the body, if not the strongest. With the sturdy structure of the skull which protects the brain from physical trauma and the blood-brain barrier which prevents the entry of microorganisms, the brain exhibits a high level of protection. However, there may be times wherein even this defense mechanism is broken down and infiltrated, like in the cases of those with poor immune systems, with the bacteria or virus able to diffuse through the blood-brain barrier and diffuse into the cerebrospinal fluid (CSF) and attacking the brain, leading to infection such as encephalitis.

During the initial stages of encephalitis, signs and symptoms of flu are usually present with fever, headache, fatigue, and sometimes cough. However, the rapid deterioration of patients with suspected encephalitis differentiates the condition from the common flu. As the infection progresses, the signature sign of encephalitis is presented which is an altered level of consciousness which can range from confusion up to fainting and maybe even coma in severe cases.

The bacteria or virus starts to attack the meninges or the brain tissue, initiating the emergency response of the body which is inflammation. The inflammatory process then activates, initiating the swelling of the brain to fight off the infection. However, this proves to be a disadvantageous event because the brain is contained within a non-expandable space which is the skull. Within the skull structure, the brain tissue, the cerebrospinal fluid (CSF), and blood are contained and maintained at a normal consistency and amount. But with the swelling of the brain tissue, the pressure within the skull increases and the circulation of blood to the brain is impeded, leading to the signs and symptoms of increased intracranial pressure to appear which may include a decreased or altered level of consciousness, confusion, weakness, elevated blood pressure, elevated temperature, a fall in pulse rate and breathing rate, and even coma.

As encephalitis progresses, other signs and symptoms also start to appear such as photophobia, behavioral changes, neck pain, nausea, vomiting, hallucinations, loss of consciousness, difficulty in swallowing, agitation, paralysis, and coma. If left untreated, the bacteria or virus may overwhelm the body's immune system, leading to an even more serious condition called "septicemia" or the generalized infection of the blood.

Brain lesions can also develop in those with encephalitis. This is brought about by destructive process caused by the infective agent, virus or bacteria, which leads to the production of abscess, neuronal dysfunction, dysfunction or destruction of the dendrites, necrosis, and infiltration of the inflammatory cells, infectious granuloma, and vasculitis.

Depending on which part of the brain is affected, signs and symptoms may present themselves as such. For example, having the occipital lobe affected may present with difficulty with vision, photophobia, and double vision, while having the frontal lobe affected may present with memory loss, speech problems, difficulty in concentration, and more.

If left untreated at its peak stage, encephalitis can cause death within 24 hours.

Diagnosing Encephalitis

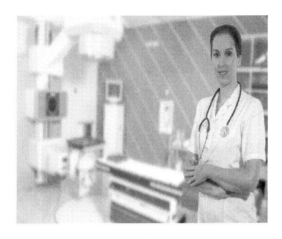

Because of how encephalitis starts with flu-like symptoms, most people can opt to delay their treatment or consultation with a physician because of mistaking it as something mild. However, the rapid progression of the disease soon alarms the patient which causes most people to seek consultation. The diagnosis of encephalitis is essential to know the progression of the disease and plan out the treatment and management options for patients with the condition. It is often difficult to diagnose encephalitis because of its mild onset and then progressing rapidly, especially since patients may opt to delay consultation because of less alarming signs and symptoms.

There are various tests that are done to confirm encephalitis which may include the following:

- **Complete blood count (CBC)**
  o CBC may show an increased white blood cell (WBC) count which indicates an active infection that is present in encephalitis.

- **Serum electrolyte levels**
  o Routine tests for serum sodium and potassium are also done to know the extent how the infection may have affected the electrolytes within the body.

- **Routine urinalysis**
  o As a standard diagnostic test in hospitals, routine urinalysis may show an increased WBC count, elevated pus cells, and bacterial cells in the urine if the infective agent came from the urinary tract.

- **Arterial blood gases (ABG)**
  ○ As the brain function may deteriorate, respiratory changes may occur and ABG can show the level of oxygen within the blood which will determine how much oxygen will be administered to the patient.

- **Gram staining, culture, and sensitivity tests of sputum, blood, urine, and other specimens**
  ○ To know the potential cause of encephalitis, gram staining and culture may be done for sputum, blood, urine, and other specimens, then sensitivity tests may be done to determine the antibiotics that can be used against the infective agent.

- **Serum creatinine**
  ○ The infection in encephalitis can become extensive and the drugs administered may cause kidney damage, as such, serum creatinine is initially

obtained to determine the function of the kidneys.

- **Electrocardiogram (ECG)**
  - Cardiac signs and symptoms like tachycardia and arrhythmia may develop due to increased ICP in encephalitis, as such; ECG is often obtained to serve as baseline data.

- **Encephalogram (EEG)**
  - An EEG is used to determine the electrical activity of the brain. In those with suspected encephalitis, EEG may show an abnormal decrease of the brain's electrical activity probably due to the infection and the swelling of the brain.

- **Lumbar puncture**
  - Being a textbook diagnostic test for those with encephalitis and meningitis, lumbar puncture or lumbar tap is used to determine the glucose and protein levels in the CSF. In lumbar puncture, CSF is acquired by using a needle that is inserted to the spinal canal and CSF is obtained. In encephalitis,

the CSF may have an increased level of protein which may indicate the presence of bacteria or virus because these microorganisms have protein-derived bodies, and a decreased level of glucose due to the bacteria or virus consuming sugar as a source of nutrients.

- **Computed Tomography scan (CT-scan)**
  o Brain imaging like CT-scan may be done in those with encephalitis to visualize possible brain abscess that may be caused by bacteria or virus. However, CT-scan is now considered only as an alternative choice when it comes to brain imaging because brain abscess is relatively uncommon in those with encephalitis and a more powerful MRI may be done.

- **Magnetic resonance imaging (MRI)**
  o Offering better resolution in visualizing the brain, MRI is done for patients with encephalitis which can show the swelling of the brain, possible brain abscess, and

the parts of the brain which are mostly affected by the infection.

- **Brain biopsy**
  - Though done rarely, brain biopsy is considered as the last leg of diagnostic test for those with encephalitis when treatments and management options aren't working. In brain biopsy, a small part of the brain tissue is obtained and the causative agent of the infection is determined.

Management of Patients with Encephalitis

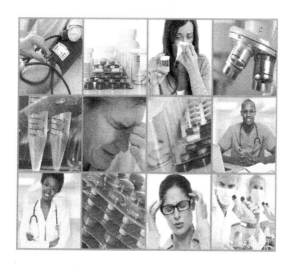

The treatment and management of patients with encephalitis is mostly symptomatic and supportive care is often done. Alleviating the symptoms is the primary goal in the treatment of this condition, so that it doesn't lead to the worsening of the infection and deterioration of the patient's condition. Once the infective agent is determined, antibiotics or antiviral agents may be administered to treat the infection. Other medications that alleviate the signs and symptoms of encephalitis may also be administered.

Pharmacologic Therapy

Medications are administered as part of the supportive care for patients with encephalitis. Drugs focus more on resolving the infection, relieving the signs and symptoms of increased ICP, relieving the inflammation, and answering the symptomatic problems with patients having encephalitis.

- **Antibiotics**
  - Once culture and sensitivity tests are done, antibiotics may be administered to relieve the active infection caused by bacteria. However, antibiotic may also be administered as part of prophylactic treatment to prevent septicemia for patients with encephalitis. Depending on the sensitivity test of the bacteria, antibiotics like cefepime, piperacillin-tazobactam, ampicillin sulbactam, ciprofloxacin, and clindamycin may be given.

- **Antiviral Agents**
  - If the cause of encephalitis is found to be a virus, antiviral agents may be given. Drugs like acyclovir and foscavir are often the choice medications when it comes to treating viral encephalitis.

- **Anti-inflammatory Agents**
  - Anti-inflammatory agents may also be given for patients with encephalitis. This aims to relieve the fever and headache as supportive care.

- **Diuretics**
  - Mannitol is an osmotic diuretic that is often given to patients with neurologic conditions such as stroke, meningitis, and encephalitis. Diuretics are used to decrease the swelling of the brain and relieve the increased ICP within the skull. As to why mannitol is the choice diuretic for neurologic conditions, that's because other diuretics like furosemide and aldactone are unable to cross the blood-brain

barrier, making these drugs incapable to decrease the swelling of the brain.

- **Anti-convulsants**
  o Seizures and muscle stiffness may be present in those with encephalitis. As such, anti-convulsant agents like phenytoin (Dilantin) may be given as a measure to relieve or prevent seizures.

- **Cerebrovascular Stimulants**
  o For neurologic conditions, cerebrovascular stimulants like citicoline are often administered to preserve the function of the brain. These drugs also promote the recovery for patients with stroke, head injuries, aneurysm, meningitis, and encephalitis.

- **Sedatives**
  o Patients with encephalitis can become irritable and restless. As such, sedatives like diazepam can be administered as part of the supportive treatment for the signs and symptoms of encephalitis

which may cause some patients to have behavioral changes, aggression, agitation, and confusion.

- **Anti-Ulcer Agents**
  - Because of the amount of drugs administered for patients with encephalitis, as well as being put on a strict nothing per orem (NPO) diet because of possible difficulty in swallowing, confusion, or unresponsiveness, anti-ulcer agents like omeprazole (Risek) and pantoprazole (Pantoloc) are often administered to prevent gastric and duodenal ulcers.

- **Other Drugs**
  - Laxatives like lactulose may be given to prevent straining when patients with encephalitis are defecating. This prevents an increase in ICP, prevents progression of headache, and prevents elevation of blood pressure.
  - Multivitamins may also be administered for these patients to support recovery, promote

appetite, and strengthen the immune system.

o Cardiac and anti-hypertensive medications such as beta blockers (e.g. propanolol, bisoprolol, atenolol), calcium channel blockers (e.g. amlodipine, nimodipine), cardiac glycosides (e.g. lanoxn), and anti-anginals (e.g. ISMN, trimetazidine), may be given as part of the supportive care and to relieve cardiac signs and symptoms in patients with encephalitis.

Supportive Care

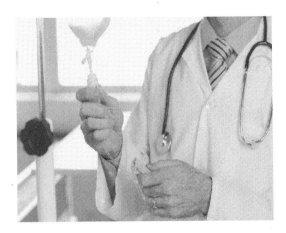

Brain Set Ablaze

Symptomatic care and supportive therapy for those with encephalitis are essential for their recovery. When it comes to encephalitis, relieving signs and symptoms is essential. Oftentimes, patients with encephalitis are put under intensive care for better monitoring of the condition, relieving signs and symptoms, and promote faster recovery. Supportive care for patients with encephalitis may include the following:

- Administration of intravenous fluids for proper hydration, providing electrolytes, and as a pathway for IV medications.
- Administration of oxygen as supplementation to provide the brain with adequate oxygen.
- Inserting a nasogastric tube (NGT) for feeding purposes if the patient is unable or has difficulty in feeding or swallowing.
- Maintaining the patient on moderate back rest to relieve increased ICP and prevent further increase of ICP.
- Inserting an indwelling catheter to monitor urine output every hour since osmotic diuretics are

administered and also to answer possible urinary incontinence.
- Putting the patient on complete bed rest to prevent increase of ICP and as a safety measure for neurologic patients who may be confused or disoriented.
- Turning the patient every 2 hours to prevent the development of pressure ulcers due to immobility in bed.
- For severe cases of encephalitis, breathing support may be provided by inserting an endotracheal tube for patients who may experience respiratory arrest.

Recovery Follow-up Therapy

Some patients who recover from encephalitis may have some neurologic deficits present. As such, follow-up therapy is often done to promote the quality of life and recover what has been lost during the course of the disease. Recovery follow-up therapy may include the following management options:

- **Speech Therapy**

o To improve muscle coordination, produce speech, and promote effective communication for those who may have experienced speech problems after recovering from encephalitis.

- **Physical Therapy**
  o To improve muscle strength, mobility, and flexibility, especially if the patient has experienced muscle weakness or paralysis of a particular limb.

- **OccupationalTherapy**
  o To promote the improvement of motor skills and relearn the everyday activities and enhance independent care for those patients who have recovered from encephalitis.

- **Psychotherapy**
  o To learn effective coping mechanisms, improve the involvement of the family in the care, and prevent the onset of depression for patients who may have neurologic deficits after recovering from encephalitis.

Prognosis

Prognosis for patients with encephalitis is generally good, provided that consultation is made early. For those patients who sought consult late wherein the signs and symptoms of encephalitis are already full-blown, it would still depend on the extent wherein the infection has done the damage, but overall, the prognosis still ranges from moderate to good. However, prognosis may be worse for patients that are included in at risk groups such as children, the elderly, and those with immuno-compromised conditions.

The signs and symptoms of encephalitis may last from a couple of days up to weeks, depending on the extent of the infection. Most cases of encephalitis are only mild, leaving with no neurological deficits after the recovery of patients. However, extensive cases of encephalitis may result in a few neurologic deficits depending on the damage that the infection may have caused. These changes may include speech problems, memory loss, personality changes, seizures, and paralysis.

Prevention of Encephalitis

While encephalitis may be a serious neurological disease, it can still be prevented. Since it's a form of infection, the primary preventive measure is to prevent the onset of infection in the first place. Minimizing contact with those who have viral infections or bacterial infections is a must, especially those who are sick, those who belong to at risk groups (children, elderly, immuno-compromised patients, undergoing chemotherapy, etc.), as well as observing strict hand washing to prevent further spread of the infection.

Fact Sheet on Encephalitis

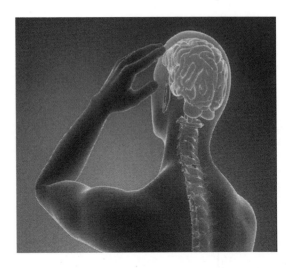

As a neurologic condition, encephalitis is often misunderstood by many people. Here are just some of the important facts about encephalitis, its causes, and its management:

- Encephalitis is often caused by a viral infection.
- Depending on the cause of encephalitis, it can be contagious.
- Vector-borne causes of encephalitis cannot be passed on from person to person as it still

needs a vector like mosquitoes or ticks to be transmitted.
- Not all people who contract the virus or bacteria that may have caused encephalitis will immediately get encephalitis; oftentimes, people who contract these viruses or bacteria don't even get sick provided that their immune system is good.
- Encephalitis may come without warning.
- Encephalitis may start out with signs and symptoms of flu like fever, headache, fatigue, and cough.
- The most prominent sign of encephalitis that you need to watch out for is a change in the level of consciousness which may lead a person to be confused, faint, or even go into a coma.
- Encephalitis is largely treatable given that it is diagnosed early.
- Diagnosis of encephalitis may be difficult because of the mild signs and symptoms it presents during its initial stage.
- Severe cases of encephalitis require hospital stay and

oftentimes, patients with encephalitis need to be taken under the intensive care unit.
- Encephalitis may last about a week, but complete recovery from the condition may range from weeks up to months.
- Mild cases of encephalitis often don't leave neurologic deficits after recovery from the disease.
- Encephalitis is largely preventable through strict hand washing and taking of vaccines against the agents that may cause it.

CONCLUSION

The brain is a fascinating piece of work. With how vital it is for the body and how strong its defense mechanism against danger, it's impressive how the brain is protected. The dense structure of the skull protects the brain from physical trauma, the cerebrospinal fluid provides additional cushion for the brain, the blood circulating to the brain contains the highest percent of oxygen and glucose which the brain utilizes everyday, and the blood-brain barrier protects the brain from numerous microorganisms and drugs that may bring harm to the brain tissue.

However, there may be cases wherein the brain is invaded by a serious type of infection. As such, something like encephalitis develops and the proper treatment and management should be done to resolve this serious disease.

Encephalitis is a serious neurological condition that starts with mild signs and symptoms, making it difficult to distinguish from a simple flu. Some people may opt to delay treatment because of this fact, but the rapid progression of the disease often leads to patients seeking immediate consultation to their attending physicians or heading to the emergency room.

The management for encephalitis mostly relies on the symptomatic management. Administering antibiotics and antiviral agents to treat the infection in encephalitis is the primary intervention done. Other interventions include supportive care through administering anti-convulsants to prevent seizures, feeding patients through a nasogastric tube for better provision of nutrients, administering anti-pyretics and anti-inflammatory agents to relieve the fever and muscle pain in encephalitis, and more.

In most cases, many patients with encephalitis recover with very good prognosis. In fact, mild cases of encephalitis leave little to no evidence of neurologic deficits upon discharge from the hospital. But severe cases of encephalitis may leave some neurologic deficits like memory loss, behavioral changes, confusion, speech problems, difficulty in swallowing, and paralysis. It's important that proper care should be given to these patients, not only during the course of the infection, but also after the infection has subsided and the patient has entered the recovery stage and follow-up therapy is essential.

While sounding life-threatening, encephalitis is a highly recoverable condition with a high number of patients being able to recover. Over the recent years, the numbers of those who have recovered from encephalitis have risen. But the most important thing here is the prevention of the infection in the first place through strict hand washing and proper hygiene habits.

As the saying goes, prevention is a more powerful tonic than the most powerful cure in the world.

Printed in Great Britain
by Amazon